# OAMAL'S ZERO POINT WEIGHT

# RECIPES COOKBOOK 2024

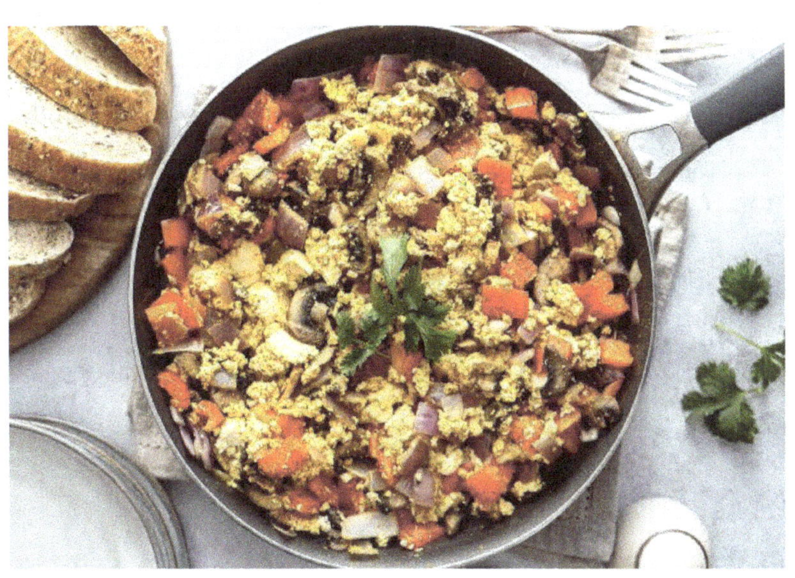

## ULTIMATE BEGINNER'S GUIDE FOR DELICIOUS

## WEIGHT MANAGEMENT – A HEALTHY LIVING

## WATCH

# CONTENTS

# INTRODUCTION

Welcome to the "Oamal's Zero Point Weight Recipes Cookbook 2024: Ultimate Beginner's Guide for Delicious Weight Management – A Healthy Living Watch"!

Embark on a transformative journey towards a healthier, more joyful lifestyle with Oamal's meticulously curated cookbook. We believe that true well-being extends beyond mere dieting; it's a harmonious blend of mindful choices, satisfying meals, and a holistic approach to living.

## The Culinary Exploration

### Zero Point Wonders:

Discover a world of culinary delights meticulously crafted by Oamal to align seamlessly with your Weight Watchers journey. From breakfast to dinner and every bite in between, Oamal's zero-point recipes redefine what's possible in the realm of flavorful, health-conscious cooking. Experience the joy of eating without the constraint of counting points, making your wellness journey both effective and enjoyable.

**Ultimate Beginner's Guide**:

Embarking on a new lifestyle can be both exciting and challenging. Oamal's cookbook serves as your compass, offering not only a diverse range of recipes but also a comprehensive beginner's guide. Dive into a wealth of information, including portion control tips, meal planning insights, and practical advice to make your transition into healthier living seamless. Whether you're new to Weight Watchers or seeking fresh inspiration, consider Oamal's cookbook your invaluable companion.

**Delicious Weight Management**:

Indulge in a feast of flavors designed by Oamal to tantalize your taste buds while supporting your health goals. Oamal firmly believes that healthy living should be a celebration of taste, and the recipes reflect this philosophy. From wholesome ingredients to innovative combinations, each dish is a testament to the idea that nutritious meals can be both satisfying and delectable.

**A Healthy Living Watch**:

Wellness extends beyond the plate and into your everyday life. Oamal's cookbook integrates a holistic approach to health, providing not just recipes but a guide to mindful living. Explore lifestyle tips, mindfulness practices, and insights into the mind-body connection. It's not just about what you eat; it's about fostering habits that contribute to a more balanced and fulfilling life.

**Savoring the Sweetness**:

In addition to Oamal's delightful recipes, clear images of each dish are included for a vivid, visual experience. Discover a guide on incorporating the natural sweetness of fruits into your routine. Understand when and how to enjoy these nature's treasures, adding a burst of freshness, nutrients, and a touch of indulgence to your daily regimen.

Are you ready to redefine your relationship with food, health, and joy? Let Oamal's "Zero Point Weight Recipes Cookbook" be your guide on this transformative journey toward a more flavorful, healthier, and joyous way of life.

# REASONS WHY EATING FRUITS FOR WEIGHT MANAGEMENT PROCESS IS ESSENTIAL

Eating fruits strategically plays a crucial role in a successful weight watchers journey. The selection, timing, and mindful consumption of fruits can contribute significantly to a balanced and effective approach to weight management.

1. **Timing and Frequency**: Distribute fruit consumption throughout the day. Consider having fruits as morning snacks to kickstart your metabolism, mid-morning or afternoon snacks for sustained energy, or as part of your main meals to enhance nutrient intake.

2. **Fiber-Focused Choices**: Prioritize fruits high in fiber, as they promote satiety and aid in digestion. Berries, apples, pears, and kiwi are excellent choices that not only add bulk to your diet but also support digestive health.

3. **Natural Sweetness for Sweet Cravings**: Fruits offer a nutritious alternative to processed sweets. Incorporating fruits into your diet can help satisfy sweet cravings while providing essential vitamins, minerals, and antioxidants.

4. **Hydration and Fullness**: Many fruits have high water content, contributing to hydration and a sense of fullness. Options like watermelon, oranges, and cantaloupe not only hydrate but also support overall well-being.

5. **Nutrient Variety**: Diversify your fruit choices to ensure a broad spectrum of nutrients. Different fruits offer unique vitamins, minerals, and antioxidants, contributing to overall health and vitality.

6. **Pre-Workout Fuel**: Some fruits, such as bananas, provide a quick and easily digestible source of energy. Consuming them before a workout can help fuel your exercise routine and support performance.

7. **Metabolism Boosters**: Certain fruits, like grapefruit, are believed to have metabolism-boosting properties. Including them in your breakfast can be a strategic choice to kickstart your metabolism for the day.

8. **Mindful Portion Control**: While fruits are nutritious, it's important to practice portion control, especially if you're closely monitoring caloric intake. Be mindful of serving sizes to avoid overconsumption, as excess calories can hinder weight management goals.

9. **Creative Meal Additions**: Experiment with incorporating fruits into various meals. Add them to salads, mix them into yogurt, or use them as toppings for whole-grain options. This not only adds flavor and variety but also increases the nutritional content of your meals.

10. **Balanced Approach**: Integrate fruits into a well-balanced diet that includes a mix of lean proteins, whole grains, and healthy fats. This ensures you meet your nutritional needs while working towards your weight management goals.

In summary, a thoughtful and intentional approach to including fruits in your diet, combined with an overall balanced lifestyle, is key to successful weight management within the framework of a weight watchers program.

# INCORPORATING FRUITS INTO A WEIGHT MANAGEMENT PLAN

1. **Bananas**: While bananas offer potassium and energy, they are higher in carbohydrates and calories. Consuming them in moderation, especially in the evening, helps manage overall calorie intake.

2. **Grapes**: Grapes are naturally sweet and can be calorie-dense. It's advisable to be mindful of portion sizes, especially during late-night snacks, to avoid excess sugar and calorie consumption.

3. **Mangoes**: Delicious but high in sugar and calories, mangoes should be enjoyed in moderation. Incorporating them sparingly helps control overall calorie intake while still benefiting from their nutritional content.

4. **Cherries**: Cherries contain natural sugars, and their sweetness can contribute to a calorie surplus. It's recommended to limit their intake, particularly if consumed close to bedtime.

5. **Pineapple**: While pineapple is rich in vitamins and minerals, it's sweet and contains natural sugars. Consuming it in moderation and preferably earlier in the day can help manage sugar intake.

6. **Dates**: Dates are calorie-dense and high in natural sugars. Being mindful of portion sizes is crucial to avoid excess calorie consumption, making them better suited for occasional treats.

7. **Watermelon**: Although hydrating, watermelon is relatively high in sugars. Moderation is key to enjoying its benefits without exceeding daily sugar intake goals.

8. **Figs**: Figs are dense in calories and natural sugars. Consuming them in controlled portions, perhaps as part of a balanced meal, helps in managing overall calorie intake.

9. **Pomegranates**: Pomegranates offer antioxidants but also contain natural sugars. Limiting their intake helps strike a balance between reaping nutritional benefits and managing sugar consumption.

10. **Lychee**: Lychees are sweet and can be high in sugars. Consuming them in moderation, such as during the morning for a natural energy boost, supports weight management goals.

11. **Raisins**: Raisins are a concentrated source of sugars and calories. Being mindful of portion sizes is essential to avoid exceeding daily calorie limits, especially when used as snacks.

12. **Kiwi**: While rich in nutrients, kiwi also contains natural sugars. Consuming them in moderation, perhaps during mid-morning or afternoon, supports a balanced diet.

13. **Papaya**: Papayas are sweet and high in natural sugars. Enjoying them in controlled amounts earlier in the day ensures better sugar management.

14. **Pears**: Pears, while healthy, are best consumed earlier in the day to aid digestion. This timing aligns with the body's natural rhythms and can support weight management.

15. **Apples**: While apples are nutritious, their natural sugar content suggests consuming them earlier in the day rather than closer to bedtime to manage overall sugar intake.

16. **Mangosteen**: Rich in antioxidants, mangosteen should be enjoyed in moderation. Including it in a balanced diet ensures the benefits without exceeding calorie and sugar goals.

17. **Persimmons**: Persimmons contain natural sugars, making them more suitable for consumption during the day when the body is more active and better able to process sugars.

18. **Guava**: While guava is a healthy choice, moderation is key due to its sugar content. Incorporating it as part of a well-balanced diet supports overall health and weight management.

19. **Dragon Fruit**: Nutrient-rich, dragon fruit is best enjoyed in controlled amounts. Including it in meals ensures a diverse range of nutrients without overwhelming sugar intake.

20. **Cantaloupe**: With its high water content, cantaloupe is hydrating. Consuming it earlier in the day aligns with natural digestion patterns and supports overall hydration and weight management.

# OAMAL'S ULTIMATE RECIPES

## 1. Zero-Point Buffalo Chicken Dip

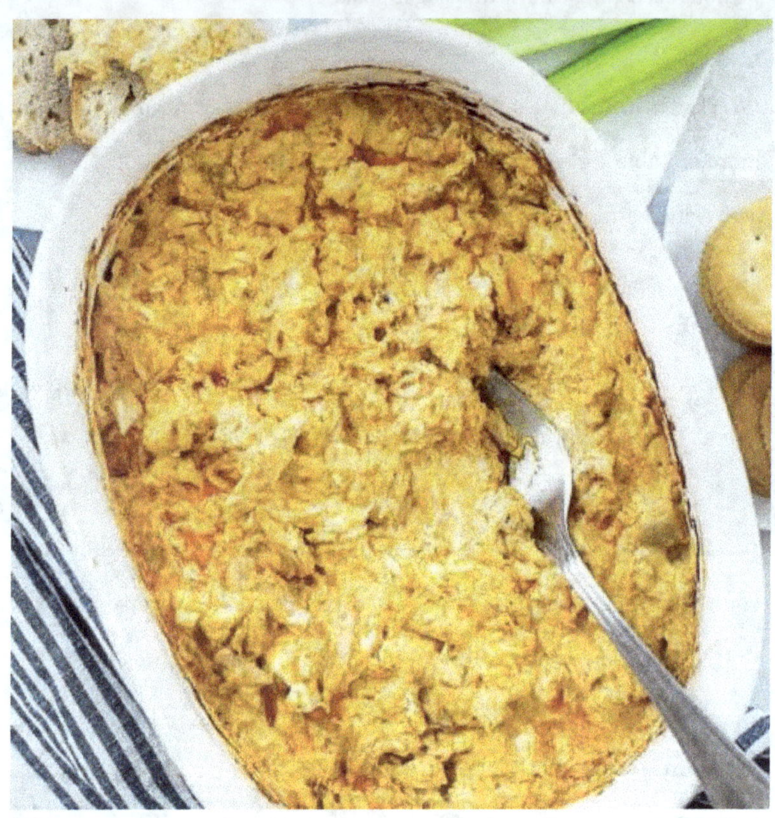

**Ingredients**:

- 2 cups shredded cooked chicken breast

- 1/2 cup fat-free Greek yogurt

- 1/2 cup hot sauce

- 1/2 cup fat-free cream cheese

- 1/2 cup shredded reduced-fat cheddar cheese

**Instructions**:

1. Preheat the oven to 350°F (175°C).

2. In a bowl, combine chicken, Greek yogurt, hot sauce, cream cheese, and cheddar cheese.

3. Transfer to a baking dish and bake until bubbly.

**Alternative Ingredients:**

Choose fat-free cream cheese for reduced fat content.

Use a mix of hot sauce and Greek yogurt for a lighter alternative.

**Reasoning:**

Fat-free cream cheese decreases overall fat while maintaining creaminess.

Greek yogurt mixed with hot sauce adds tanginess without extra calories.

**Nutritional Information (per serving):**

Calories: 120.      Protein: 15g      Carbohydrates: 4g.      Fat: 3g

<h1 style="text-align:center">2. Zero-Point Banana Pancakes</h1>

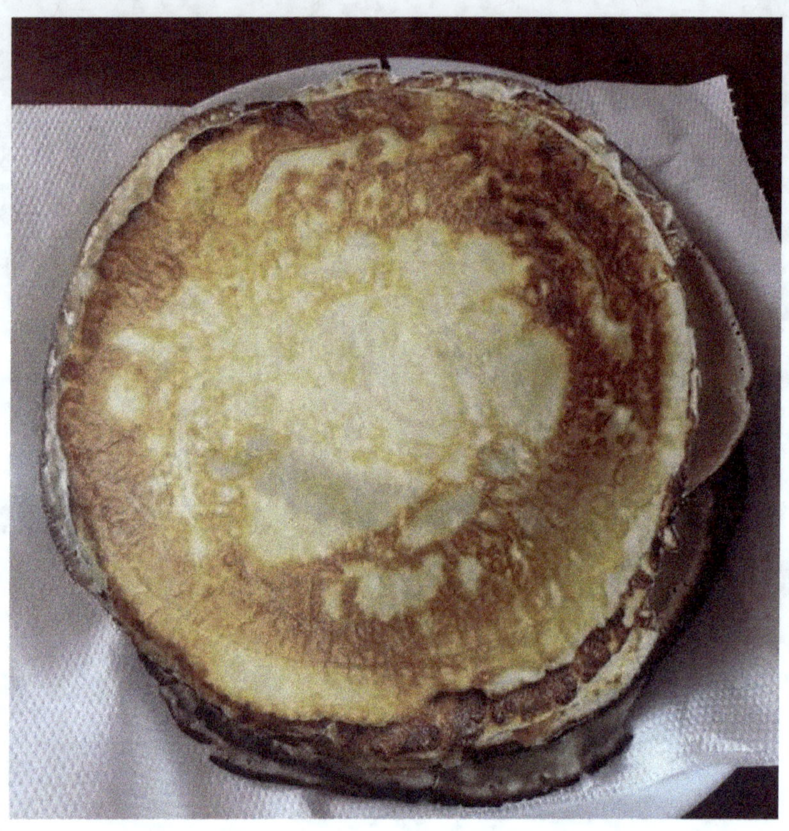

**Ingredients**:

- 2 ripe bananas

- 2 eggs

- 1/2 teaspoon baking powder

- Pinch of salt

- Optional: vanilla extract

**Instructions:**

1. Mash bananas in a bowl.

2. Add eggs, baking powder, and salt. Mix well.

3. Heat a non-stick pan over medium heat.

4. Pour small amounts of batter onto the pan.

5. Cook until bubbles form, then flip and cook the other side.

**Alternative Ingredients:**

Substitute regular eggs with egg whites for lower cholesterol.

Use whole wheat flour instead of all-purpose flour for added fiber.

**Reasoning:**

Egg whites reduce calories and cholesterol, making the recipe even healthier.

Whole wheat flour adds more nutrients and fiber, promoting satiety.

**Nutritional Information (per serving):**

Calories: 150.      Protein: 8g.      Carbohydrates: 30g

Fiber: 4g.          Fat: 1g

**3. Zero-Point Onion Dip**

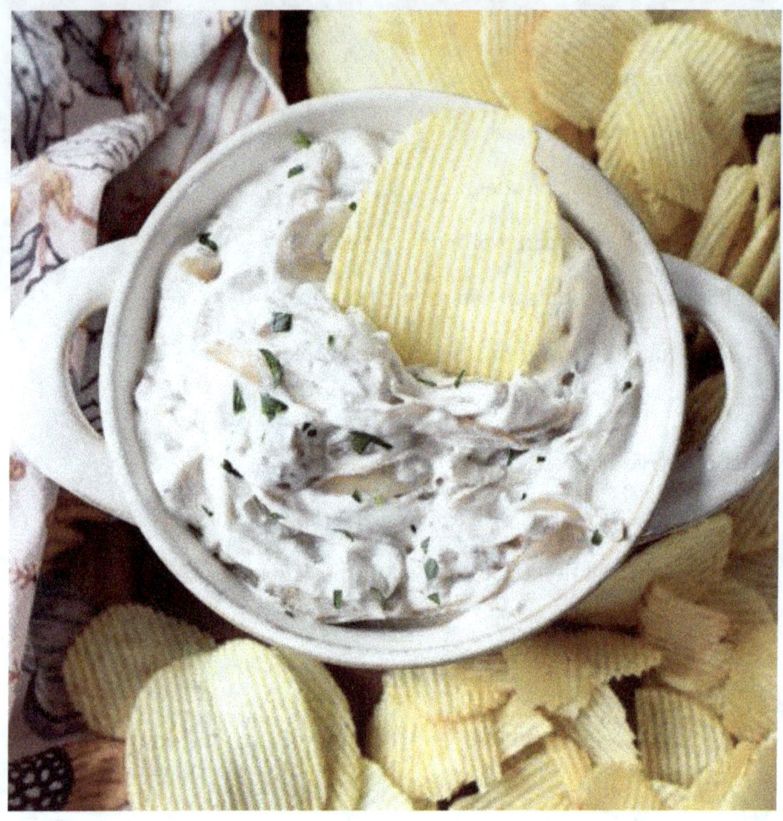

**Ingredients**:

- 2 cups fat-free Greek yogurt

- 1 onion, finely chopped - 1 teaspoon onion powder

- 1 teaspoon garlic powder - Salt and pepper to taste

**Instructions**:

1. Mix Greek yogurt, chopped onion, onion powder, and garlic powder in a bowl.

2. Season with salt and pepper.

3. Refrigerate for at least an hour before serving.

**Alternative Ingredients:**

Opt for fat-free sour cream instead of Greek yogurt.

Use a mix of fresh herbs like chives and parsley for added flavor.

Eat with any of your chips choice, e.g, Potato chips.

**Reasoning:**

Fat-free sour cream maintains the creamy texture with fewer calories.

Fresh herbs enhance the taste without added points.

**Nutritional Information (per serving):**

Calories: 40

Protein: 2g

Carbohydrates: 6g

Fat: 0g

# 4. Amazing Zero-Point Deviled Eggs

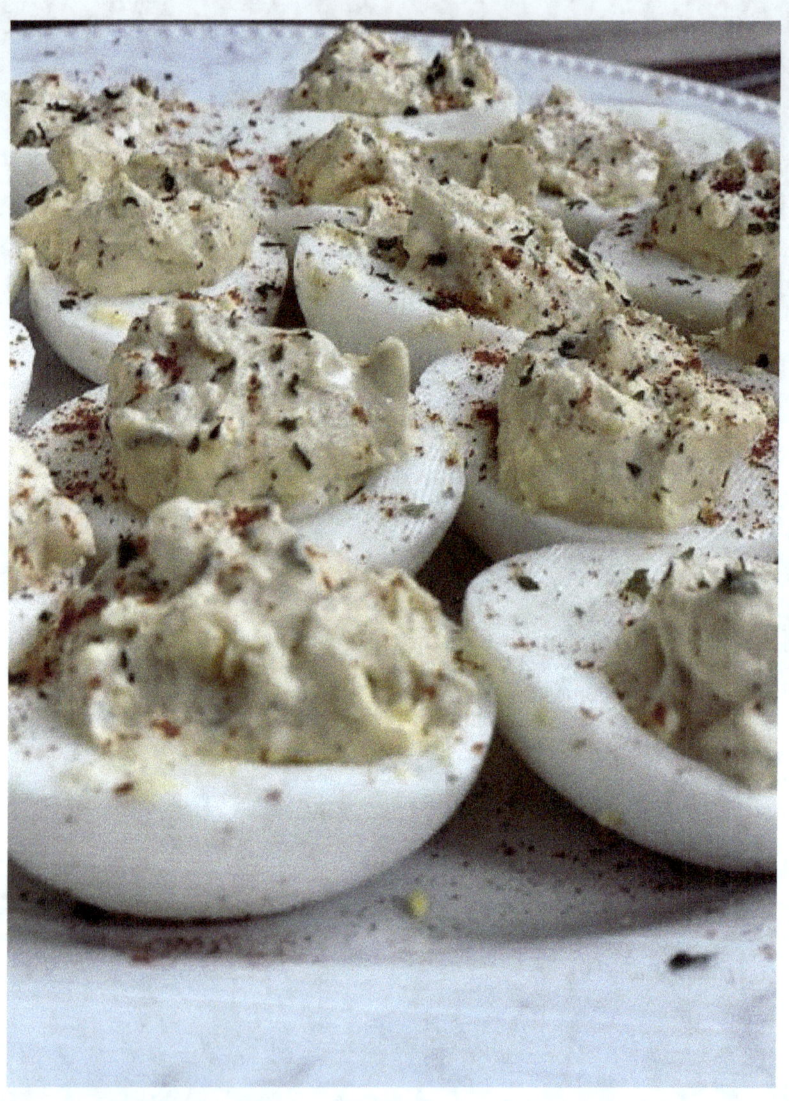

**Ingredients**:

- 6 hard-boiled eggs - 1/4 cup fat-free Greek yogurt

- 1 tablespoon Dijon mustard

- Salt and pepper to taste - Paprika for garnish


**Instructions**:

1. Cut boiled eggs in half; remove yolks and place in a bowl.

2. Mix yolks with Greek yogurt, mustard, salt, and pepper.

3. Spoon mixture back into egg whites.

4. Sprinkle it with paprika.


**Alternative Ingredients:**

Replace regular mayo with fat-free mayo or Greek yogurt.

Use Dijon mustard for added flavor without additional points.


**Reasoning:**

Fat-free mayo or Greek yogurt reduces fat content.

Dijon mustard provides a zesty kick without added calories.


**Nutritional Information (per serving, 2 halves):**

Calories: 50.     Protein: 6g.     Carbohydrates: 1g.     Fat: 3g

# 5. Tofu Scramble

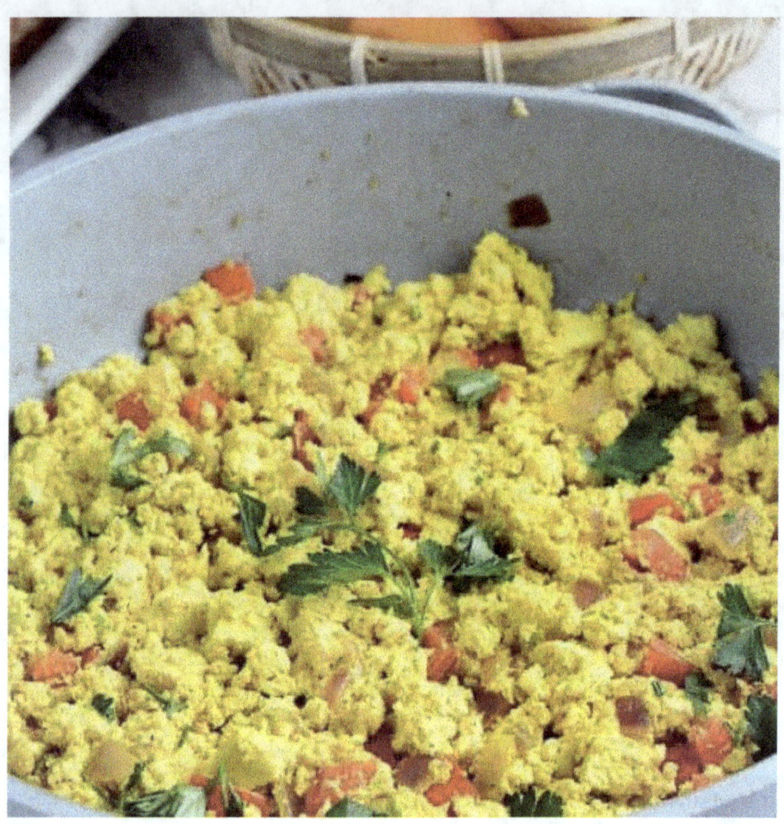

**Ingredients**:

- 1 block firm tofu, crumbled

- 1 tablespoon olive oil

- 1 bell pepper, diced

- 1 onion, diced

- 1 teaspoon turmeric

- Salt and pepper to taste

## Instructions:

1. Heat oil in a pan, sauté onion and bell pepper until softened.

2. Add crumbled tofu, turmeric, salt, and pepper.

3. Cook until tofu is heated through.

## Alternative Ingredients:

Opt for extra-firm tofu for a heartier texture.

Use a mix of colorful bell peppers for added nutrients.

## Reasoning:

Extra-firm tofu enhances the chewiness of the scramble.

Bell peppers add vitamins and a vibrant appearance.

## Nutritional Information (per serving):

Calories: 120

Protein: 15g

Carbohydrates: 6g

Fat: 5g

## 6. Zero-Point Chili

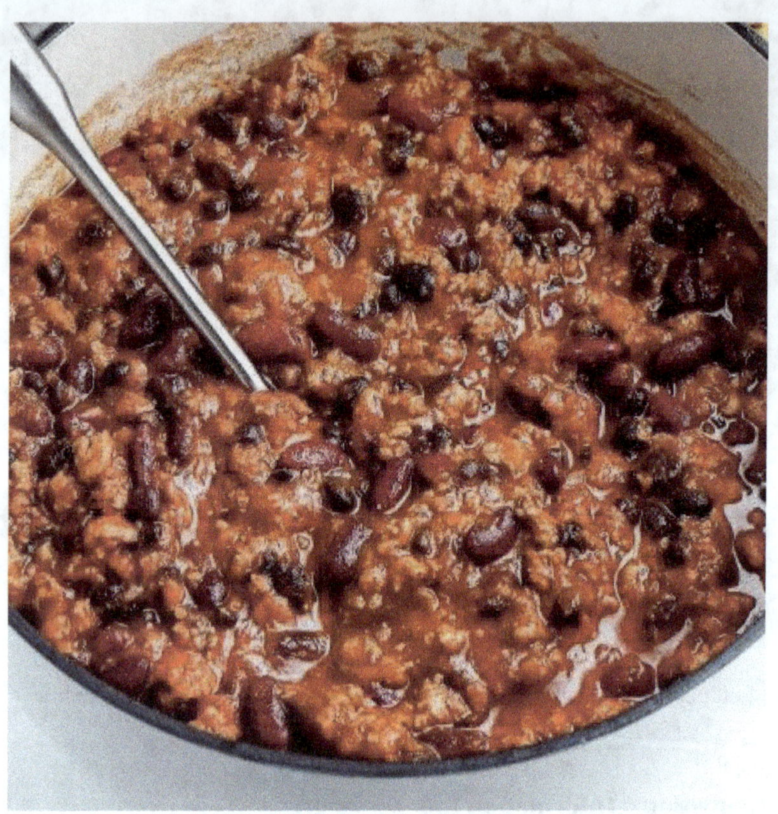

**Ingredients**:

- 1 lb lean ground turkey - 1 onion, diced - 2 cloves garlic, minced

- 1 can (15 oz) black beans, drained and rinsed

- 1 can (15 oz) kidney beans, drained and rinsed

- 1 can (15 oz) diced tomatoes

- 1 cup frozen corn - 1 tablespoon chili powder

- 1 teaspoon cumin - Salt and pepper to taste

**Instructions**:

1. In a large pot, cook ground turkey until browned.

2. Add onion and garlic; cook until softened.

3. Add beans, tomatoes, corn, chili powder, cumin, salt, and pepper.

4. Simmer for at least 30 minutes.

**Alternative Ingredients:**

Use ground chicken or turkey instead of beef for a leaner option.

Incorporate a variety of beans like black beans, kidney beans, and pinto beans for added fiber.

**Reasoning:**

Lean poultry reduces saturated fat content.

A mix of beans provides a range of nutrients and boosts fiber.

**Nutritional Information (per serving):**

| Calories: 200 | Protein: 20g | |
| --- | --- | --- |
| Carbohydrates: 25g. | Fiber: 8g. | Fat: 5g |

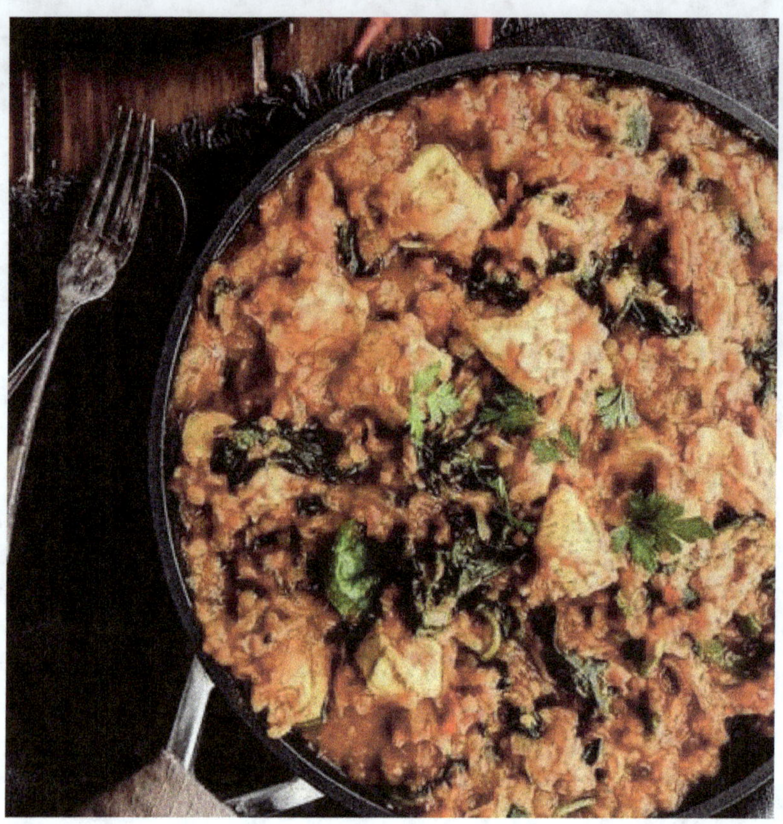

**Ingredients**:

- 1 lb boneless, skinless chicken breast, cubed

- 1 onion, chopped - 2 cloves garlic, minced

- 1 can (15 oz) tomato sauce - 1 cup fat-free chicken broth

- 1 tablespoon curry powder

- 1 teaspoon cumin

- Salt and pepper to taste

**Instructions**:

1. In a skillet, cook chicken until browned.

2. Add onion and garlic; cook until softened.

3. Stir in tomato sauce, chicken broth, curry powder, cumin, salt, and

pepper.

4. Simmer until chicken is cooked through.

**Alternative Ingredients:**

Choose boneless, skinless chicken thighs for more flavor.

Use coconut milk or almond milk for a dairy-free alternative.

**Reasoning:**

Chicken thighs add richness and depth of flavor.

Coconut or almond milk provides creaminess without dairy.

**Nutritional Information (per serving):**

Calories: 250.                    Protein: 22g

Carbohydrates: 10g.          Fat: 15g

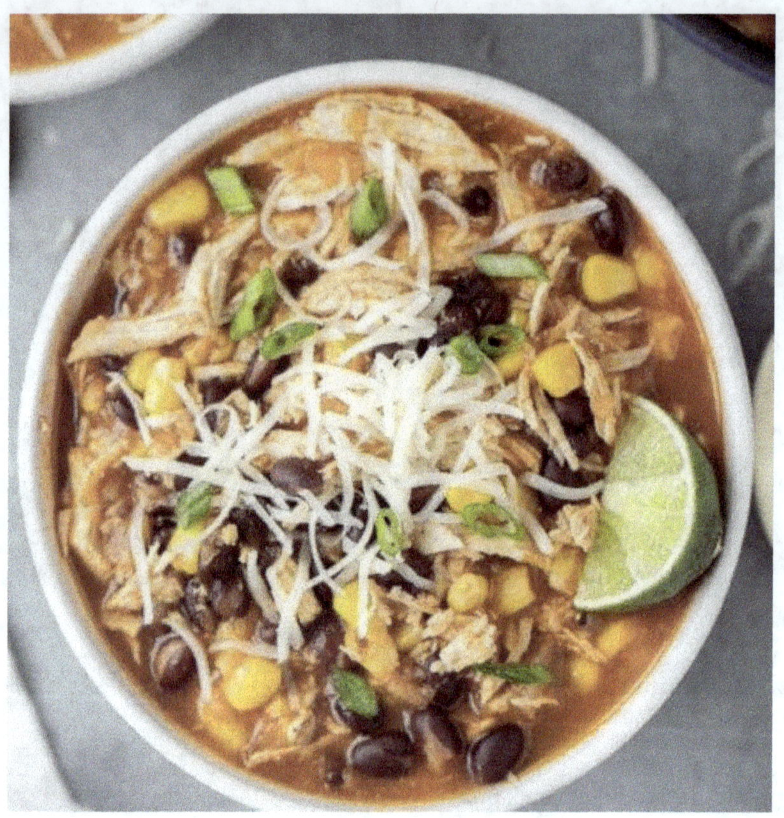

**Ingredients**:

- 1 lb boneless, skinless chicken breast, shredded

- 1 can (15 oz) black beans, drained and rinsed

- 1 can (15 oz) corn, drained

- 1 can (15 oz) diced tomatoes

- 1 packet taco seasoning - 1 cup fat-free chicken broth

- Optional toppings: cilantro, lime, shredded lettuce

**Instructions**:

1. In a large pot, combine chicken, black beans, corn, tomatoes, taco seasoning, and chicken broth.

2. Simmer until heated through.

3. Serve with optional toppings.

**Alternative Ingredients:**

Opt for lean ground turkey instead of chicken.

Use low-sodium vegetable broth for a lighter option.

**Reasoning:**

Lean ground turkey reduces saturated fat.

Low-sodium vegetable broth helps control sodium intake.

**Nutritional Information (per serving):**

Calories: 180

Protein: 18g

Carbohydrates: 20g

Fat: 4g

# 9. Zero Point Salsa Chicken

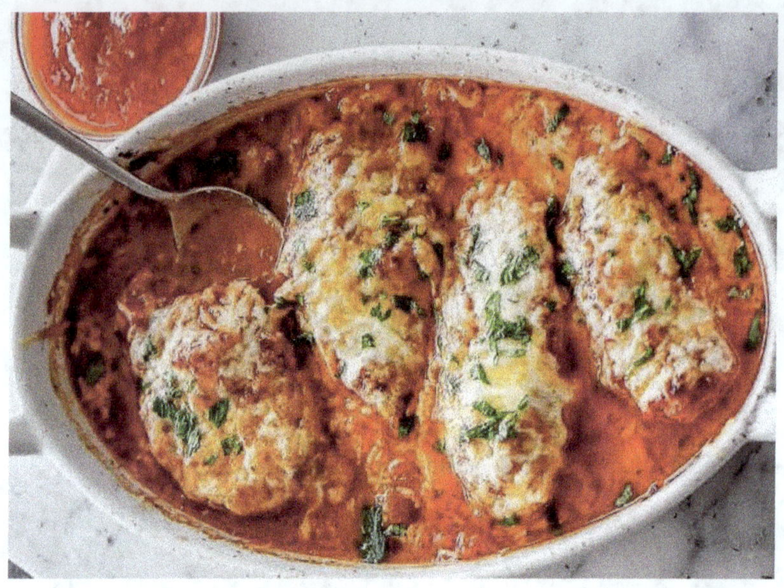

**Ingredients**:

- 4 boneless, skinless chicken breasts

- 1 cup salsa

- 1 teaspoon cumin

- 1 teaspoon garlic powder

- 1 teaspoon onion powder

- Salt and pepper to taste

**Instructions**:

1. Preheat the oven to 375°F (190°C).

2. Place chicken breasts in a baking dish.

3. Season with cumin, garlic powder, onion powder, salt, and pepper.

4. Pour salsa over chicken.

5. Bake until chicken is cooked through.

## Alternative Ingredients:

Choose boneless, skinless chicken thighs for more flavor.

Make homemade salsa using fresh tomatoes, onions, and cilantro.

## Reasoning:

Chicken thighs add richness and succulence.

Fresh homemade salsa ensures minimal added sugars.

## Nutritional Information (per serving):

Calories: 220

Protein: 24g

Carbohydrates: 10g

Fat: 10g

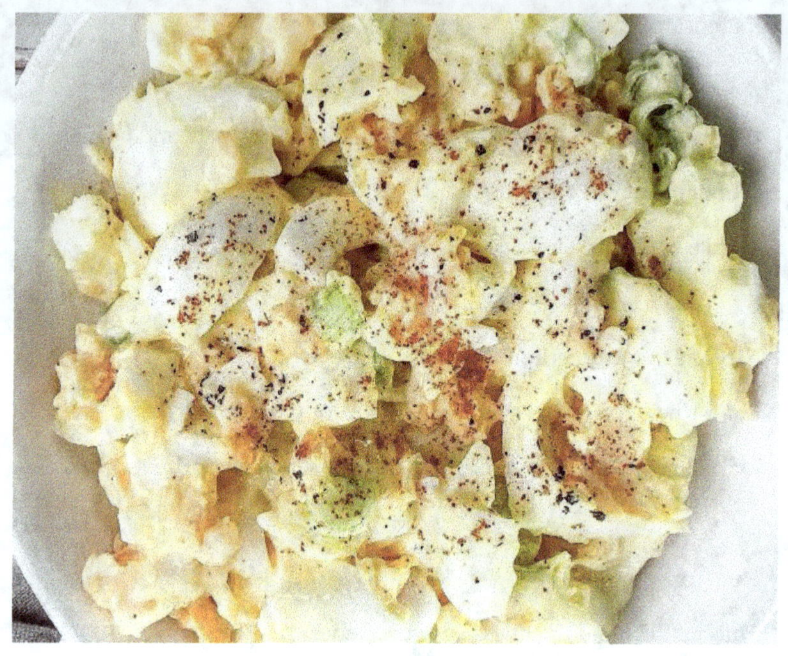

**Ingredients**:

- 6 hard-boiled eggs, chopped

- 1/2 cup fat-free Greek yogurt

- 2 teaspoons Dijon mustard

- 1 tablespoon fresh dill, chopped

- Salt and pepper to taste

**Instructions**:

1. In a bowl, combine chopped eggs, Greek yogurt, Dijon mustard, dill, salt, and pepper.

2. Mix until well combined.

3. Refrigerate before serving.

## Alternative Ingredients:

Use fat-free Greek yogurt instead of mayo.

Add chopped celery and bell peppers for extra crunch and nutrients.

## Reasoning:

Fat-free Greek yogurt reduces overall fat content.

Celery and bell peppers add texture and vitamins.

## Nutritional Information (per serving):

Calories: 100

Protein: 12g

Carbohydrates: 5g

Fat: 3g

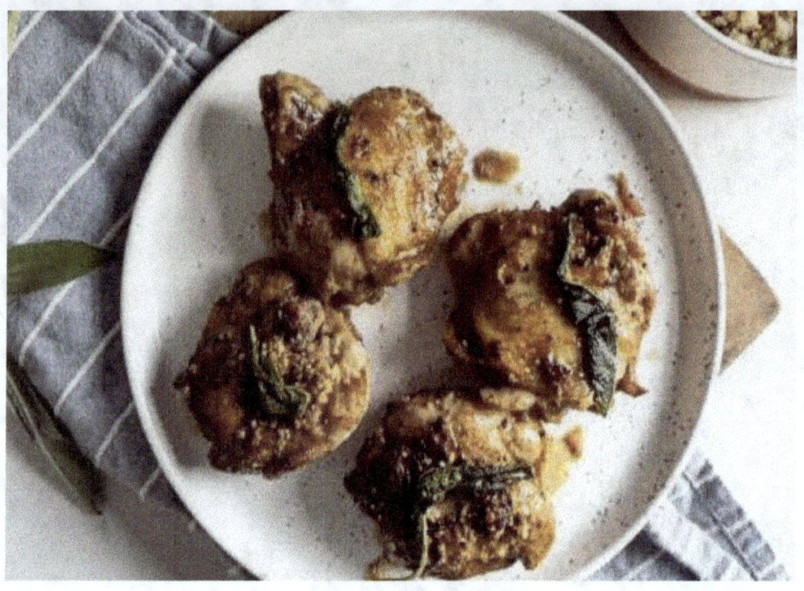

**Ingredients**:

- 4 boneless, skinless chicken breasts

- 2 tablespoons fresh sage, chopped

- 2 tablespoons unsalted butter

- Salt and pepper to taste

- Lemon wedges for serving

**Instructions**:

1. Season chicken breasts with salt and pepper.

2. Grill until cooked through.

3. In a small pan, melt butter and add chopped sage.

4. Pour sage butter over grilled chicken.

5. Serve with lemon wedges.

**Alternative Ingredients:**

Use boneless, skinless chicken thighs for a juicier option.

Substitute unsalted ghee for butter for a rich flavor with less saturated fat.

**Reasoning:**

Chicken thighs offer more moisture and flavor.

Ghee provides a buttery taste with reduced saturated fat.

**Nutritional Information (per serving):**

Calories: 250

Protein: 25g

Carbohydrates: 0g

Fat: 16g

## 12. Weight Watchers Zero-Point Cheesecake

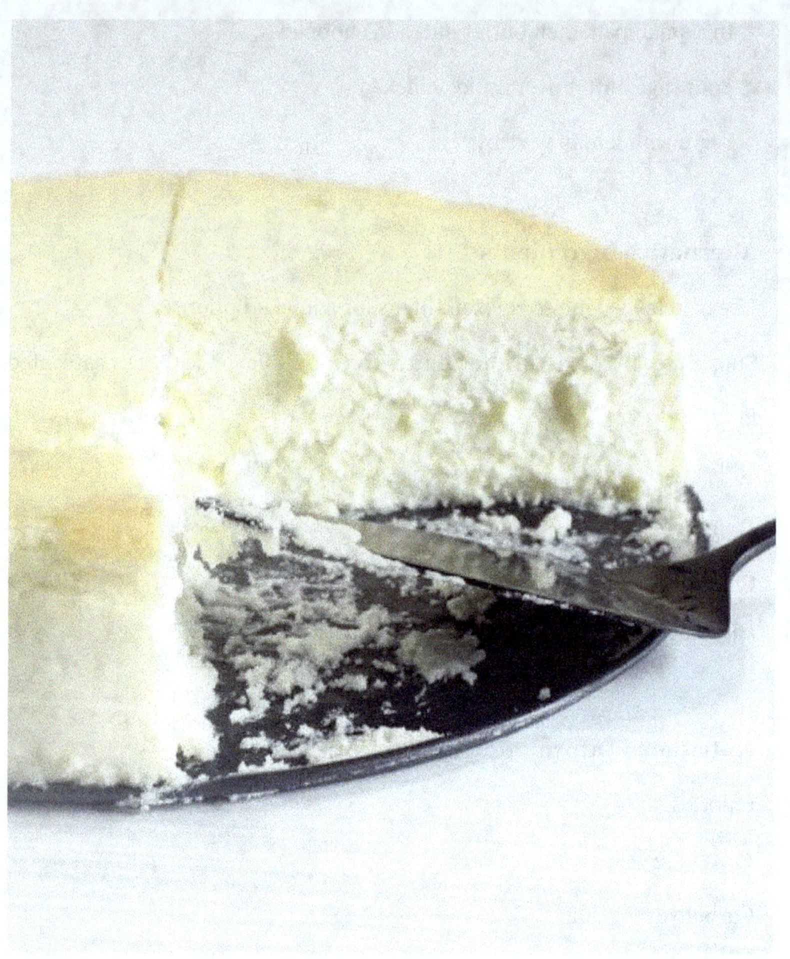

**Ingredients:**

- 2 cups fat-free Greek yogurt

- 2 packages sugar-free Jello (any flavor)

- 1 teaspoon vanilla extract - 1/2 cup boiling water

**Instructions**:

1. In a bowl, mix Greek yogurt and vanilla extract.

2. Dissolve Jello in boiling water; let it cool slightly.

3. Gradually add Jello mixture to the yogurt, stirring continuously.

4. Pour into a dish and refrigerate until set.

**Alternative Ingredients:**

Opt for fat-free cream cheese and Greek yogurt.

Use sugar substitutes like stevia or erythritol.

**Reasoning:**

Fat-free dairy products reduce overall fat content.

Sugar substitutes cut down on added sugars.

**Nutritional Information (per serving):**

Calories: 120

Protein: 8g

Carbohydrates: 10g

Fat: 4g

# 13. Spiced Coffee Custards

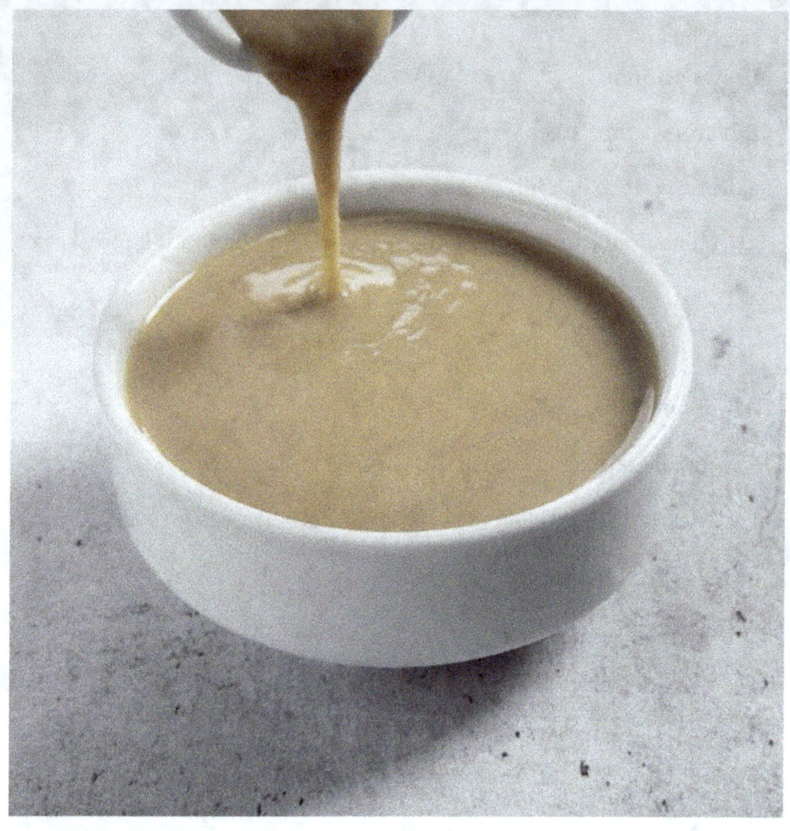

**Ingredients**:

- 2 cups black coffee, cooled

- 1 cup fat-free milk

- 4 eggs

- 1/2 cup sweetener (stevia or your preference)

- 1 teaspoon ground cinnamon

- 1/2 teaspoon ground nutmeg

**Instructions**:

1. Preheat the oven to 325°F (163°C).

2. In a bowl, whisk together coffee, milk, eggs, sweetener, cinnamon, and nutmeg.

3. Pour into custard cups and bake in a water bath until set.

**Alternative Ingredients:**

Choose almond milk or coconut milk for a dairy-free option.

Use a sugar substitute for sweetness.

**Reasoning:**

Dairy-free milk alternatives cater to dietary restrictions.

Sugar substitute reduces added sugars.

**Nutritional Information (per serving):**

Calories: 80

Protein: 4g

Carbohydrates: 10g

Fat: 3g

# 14. Weight Watchers Zero-Point Banana Nice Cream

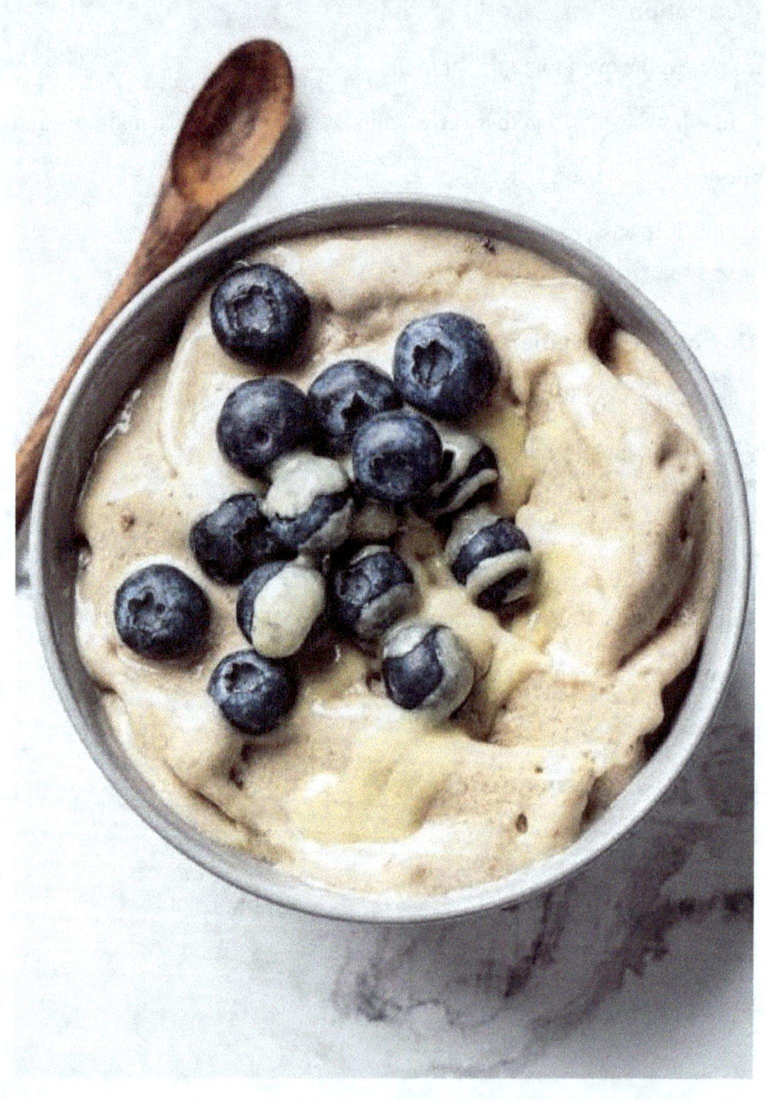

**Ingredients**:

- 4 ripe bananas, frozen

- 1 teaspoon vanilla extract

- Optional: toppings like berries or nuts


**Instructions**:

1. Blend frozen bananas and vanilla extract until smooth.

2. Serve immediately as a healthy ice cream alternative.

3. Top with berries or nuts if desired.


**Alternative Ingredients:**

Add a handful of spinach for added nutrients and a vibrant green color.

Include a tablespoon of almond butter for a nutty flavor.


**Reasoning:**

Spinach enhances nutritional content without altering taste.

Almond butter adds healthy fats and depth of flavor.


**Nutritional Information (per serving):**

| | |
|---|---|
| Calories: 150. | Protein: 2g |
| Carbohydrates: 35g. | Fat: 5g |

# 15. Southwestern Chicken Skillet

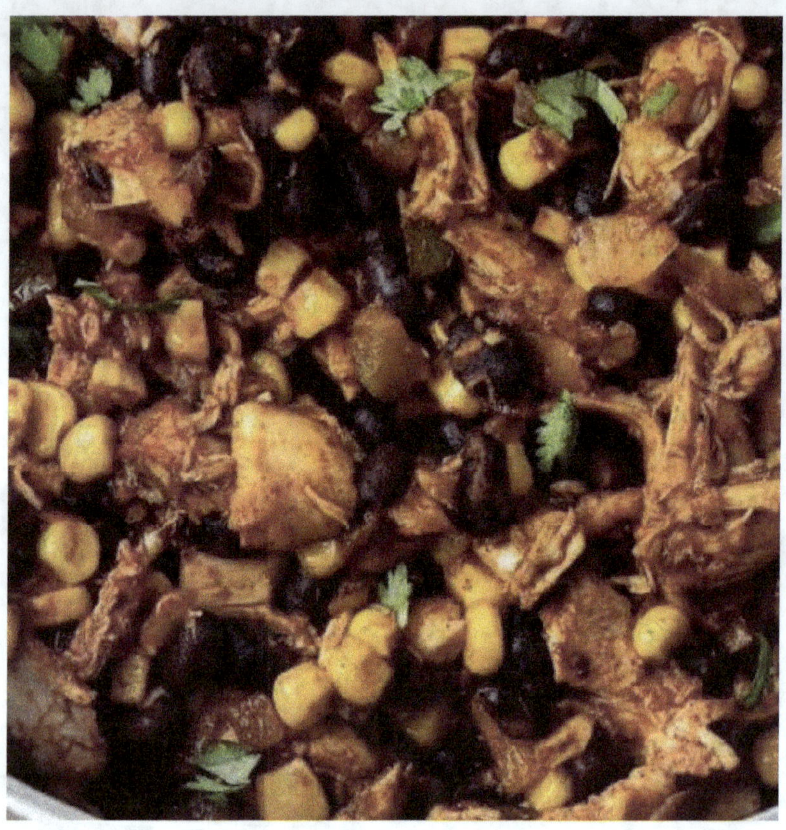

**Ingredients**:

- 1 lb boneless, skinless chicken breast, diced

- 1 bell pepper, sliced - 1 onion, sliced

- 1 can (15 oz) black beans, drained and rinsed

- 1 cup corn kernels

- 1 tablespoon chili powder

- 1 teaspoon cumin - Salt and pepper to taste

## Instructions:

1. In a skillet, cook chicken until browned.

2. Add bell pepper, onion, black beans, corn, chili powder, cumin, salt, and pepper.

3. Cook until vegetables are tender and chicken is cooked through.

## Alternative Ingredients:

Use lean ground turkey for a lighter option.

Opt for quinoa instead of rice for added protein and fiber.

## Reasoning:

Lean ground turkey reduces saturated fat.

Quinoa provides more protein and fiber than traditional rice.

## Nutritional Information (per serving):

Calories: 300

Protein: 25g

Carbohydrates: 25g

Fat: 10g

# 16. Lentil & Corn Chili

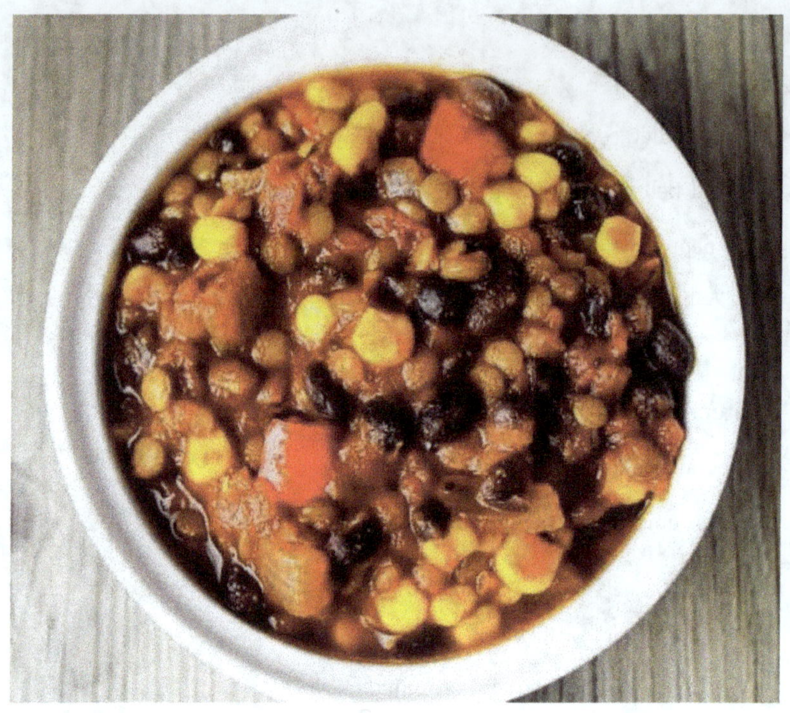

**Ingredients**:

- 1 cup dry lentils, rinsed

- 1 can (15 oz) corn, drained

- 1 can (15 oz) diced tomatoes

- 1 onion, diced

- 2 cloves garlic, minced

- 1 tablespoon chili powder

- 1 teaspoon cumin

- Salt and pepper to taste

**Instructions**:

1. In a pot, combine lentils, corn, tomatoes, onion, garlic, chili powder, cumin, salt, and pepper.

2. Cover with water and simmer until lentils are tender.

**Alternative Ingredients:**

Use red lentils for quicker cooking.

Substitute lean ground turkey for a lighter option.

Opt black bean

**Reasoning:**

Red lentils cook faster than regular lentils.

Lean ground turkey reduces overall fat content.

**Nutritional Information (per serving):**

Calories: 220

Protein: 18g.   Carbohydrates: 30g

Fiber: 8g

Fat: 5g

# 17. Double Chocolate Mug Muffin

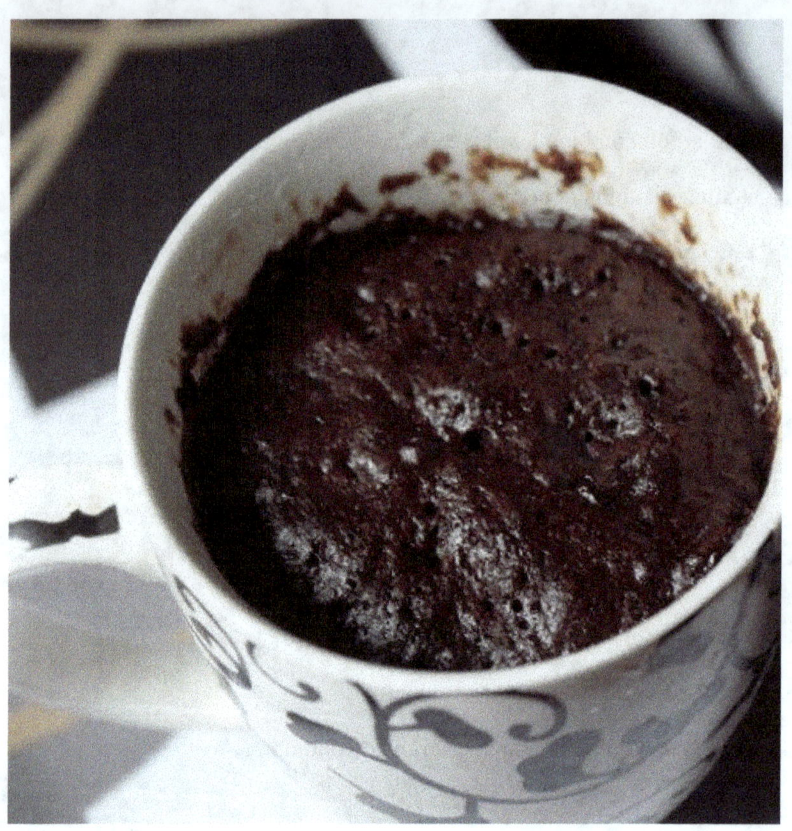

**Ingredients:**

- 3 tablespoons flour

- 2 tablespoons unsweetened cocoa powder

- 1 tablespoon sweetener (stevia or your preference)

- 1/4 teaspoon baking powder

- Pinch of salt

- 3 tablespoons fat-free milk

- 1/2 teaspoon vanilla extract

**Instructions**:

1. In a mug, whisk together flour, cocoa powder, sweetener, baking powder, and salt.

2. Add milk and vanilla extract; stir until smooth.

3. Microwave for 1-2 minutes until set.

**Alternative Ingredients:**

Use almond flour for a gluten-free option.

Choose a sugar substitute for sweetness.

**Reasoning:**

Almond flour provides a gluten-free alternative.

Sugar substitute reduces added sugars.

**Nutritional Information (per serving):**

| | |
|---|---|
| Calories: 180. | Protein: 7g |
| Carbohydrates: 15g. | Fat: 12g |

# 18. Yogurt Chicken

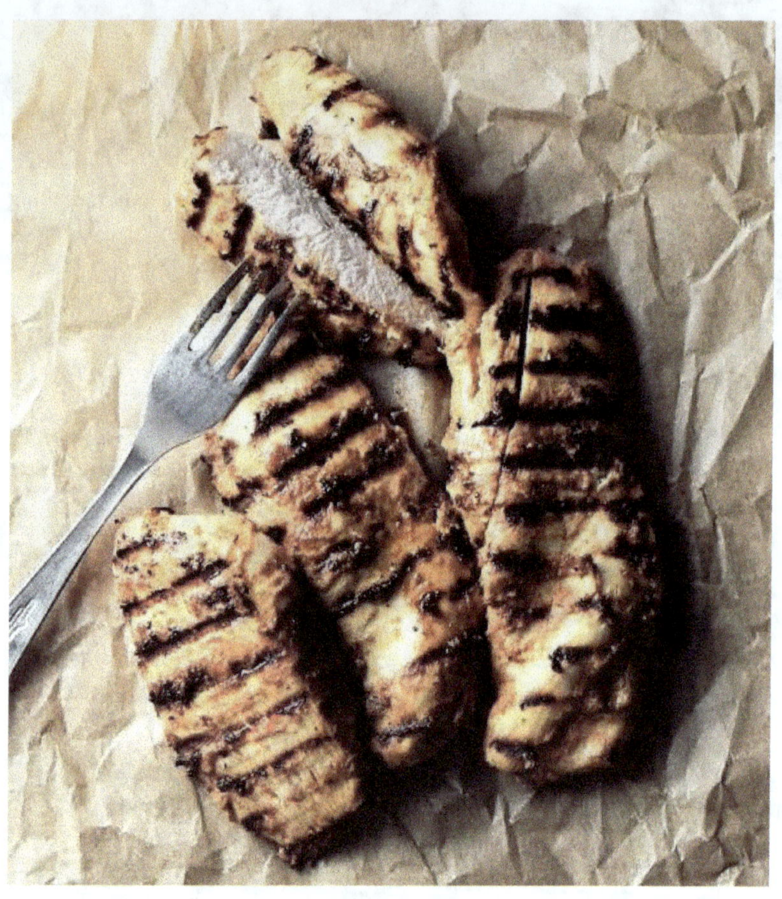

**Ingredients**:

- 4 boneless, skinless chicken breasts

- 1 cup fat-free Greek yogurt

- 1 tablespoon garlic powder

- 1 tablespoon onion powder

- 1 teaspoon paprika

- Salt and pepper to taste

**Instructions**:

1. Preheat oven to 375°F (190°C).

2. Mix Greek yogurt, garlic powder, onion powder, paprika, salt, and pepper.

3. Coat chicken breasts with the yogurt mixture.

4. Bake until chicken is cooked through.

**Alternative Ingredients:**

Use fat-free Greek yogurt instead of regular yogurt.

Substitute chicken breasts for a leaner cut.

**Reasoning:**

Fat-free Greek yogurt reduces overall fat content.

Chicken breasts provide lean protein.

**Nutritional Information (per serving):**

Calories: 220.

Protein: 30g

Carbohydrates: 5g.

Fat: 8g

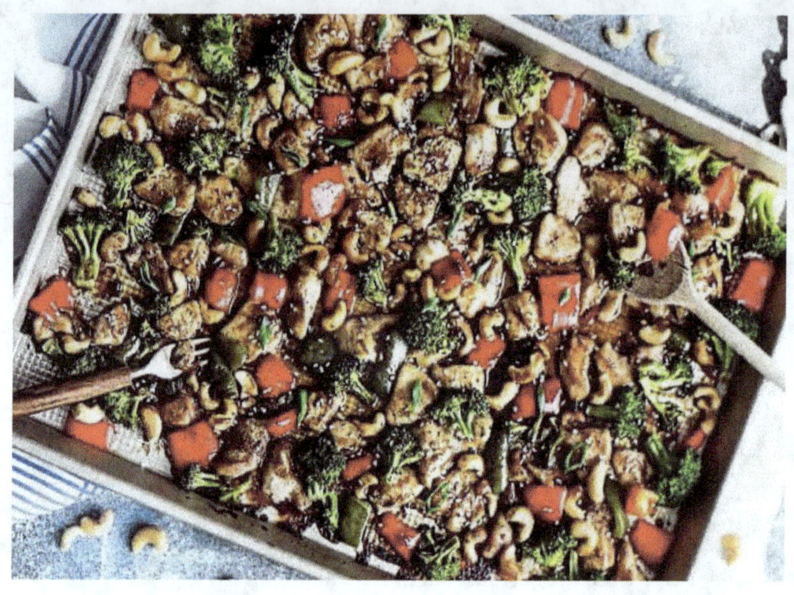

**Ingredients**:

- 1 lb boneless, skinless chicken thighs

- 1 cup broccoli florets

- 1 bell pepper, sliced

- 1/2 cup cashews

- 2 tablespoons soy sauce

- 1 tablespoon rice vinegar

- 1 teaspoon ginger, grated

**Instructions**:

1. Preheat oven to 400°F (200°C).

2. Place chicken, broccoli, bell pepper, and cashews on a baking sheet.

3. Mix soy sauce, rice vinegar, and ginger; pour over the chicken and vegetables.

4. Bake until chicken is cooked through.

**Alternative Ingredients:**

Use skinless chicken thighs for more flavor.

Opt for unsalted cashews for lower sodium.

**Reasoning:**

Skinless chicken thighs add richness without the skin.

Unsalted cashews help control sodium intake.

**Nutritional Information (per serving):**

Calories: 300

Protein: 25g

Carbohydrates: 15g

Fat: 15g

# 20. Cilantro Lime Dressing

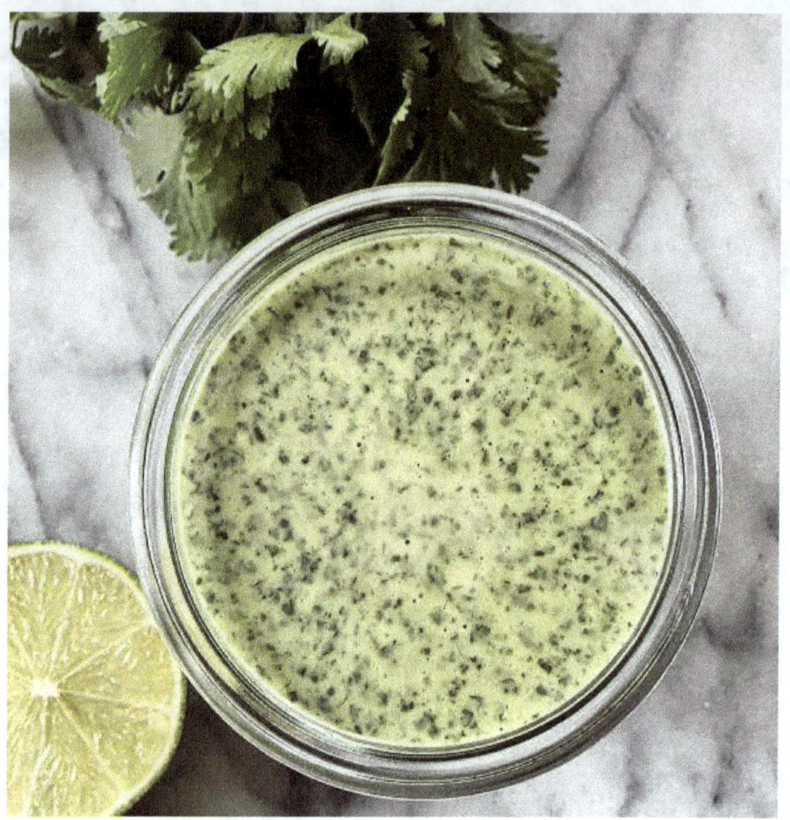

**Ingredients**:

- 1/2 cup fat-free Greek yogurt

- 1/4 cup lime juice

- 2 tablespoons fresh cilantro, chopped

- 1 teaspoon honey

- Salt and pepper to taste

**Instructions**:

1. In a bowl, whisk together Greek yogurt, lime juice, cilantro, honey, salt, and pepper.

2. Use as a dressing for salads or grilled chicken.

## Alternative Ingredients:

Choose fat-free Greek yogurt instead of regular yogurt.

Use agave nectar or a sugar substitute for sweetness.

## Reasoning:

Fat-free Greek yogurt reduces overall fat content.

Agave nectar or a sugar substitute cuts down on added sugars.

## Nutritional Information (per serving):

Calories: 40

Protein: 2g

Carbohydrates: 5g

Fat: 0g

## 21. Sweet Potato & Chicken Patties

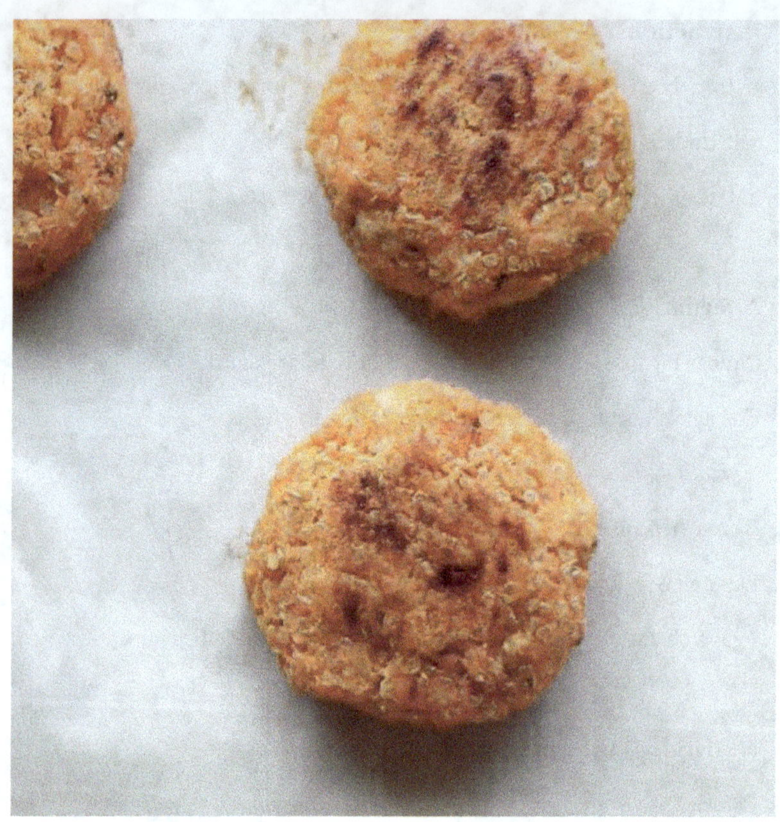

**Ingredients**:

- 1 lb ground chicken

- 2 cups sweet potatoes, grated

- 1 onion, finely chopped

- 2 cloves garlic, minced

- 1 teaspoon paprika

- Salt and pepper to taste

- 2 tablespoons olive oil (for cooking)

**Instructions**:

1. In a bowl, combine ground chicken, sweet potatoes, onion, garlic, paprika, salt, and pepper.

2. Form mixture into patties.

3. Heat olive oil in a skillet and cook patties until browned on both sides.

**Alternative Ingredients:**

Use ground chicken breast for a leaner option.

Opt for whole wheat breadcrumbs for added fiber.

**Reasoning:**

Ground chicken breast reduces saturated fat.

Whole wheat breadcrumbs add more fiber.

**Nutritional Information (per serving):**

Calories: 220.

Protein: 25g

Carbohydrates: 15g.

Fiber: 3g

Fat: 8g

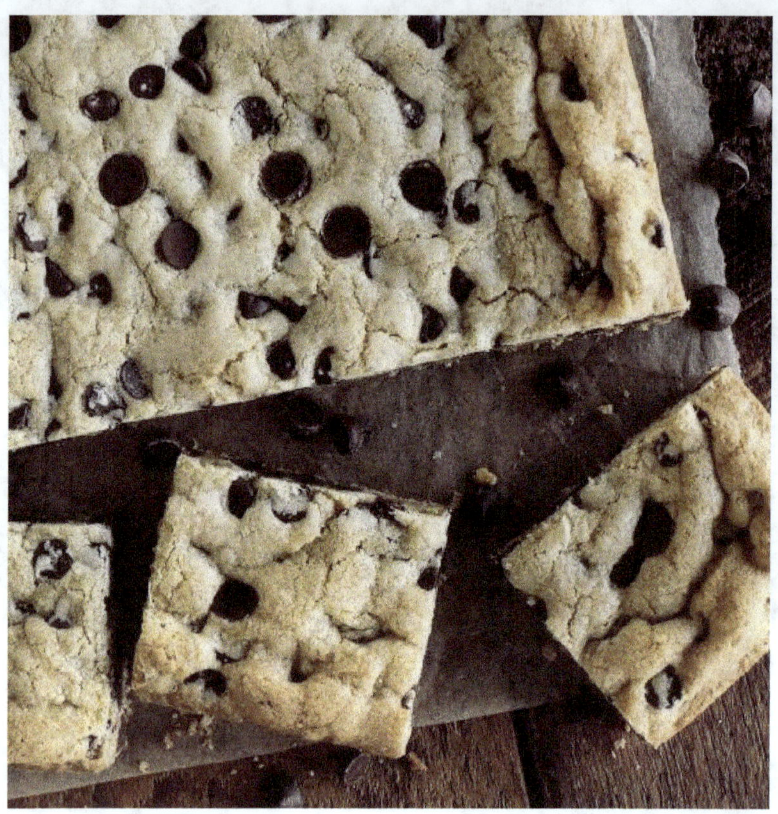

**Ingredients:**

- 2 ripe bananas, mashed

- 1/2 cup unsweetened applesauce

- 1 cup rolled oats

- 1/4 cup almond flour

- 1/4 cup mini chocolate chips

- 1 teaspoon vanilla extract

**Instructions**:

1. Preheat the oven to 350°F (175°C).

2. Mix mashed bananas, applesauce, oats, almond flour, chocolate chips,

and vanilla extract.

3. Spread mixture in a baking dish.

4. Bake until golden brown.

**Alternative Ingredients:**

Choose almond flour for a gluten-free option.

Use dark chocolate chips for a richer flavor with less sugar.

**Reasoning:**

Almond flour provides a gluten-free alternative.

Dark chocolate chips contain less sugar and more antioxidants.

**Nutritional Information (per serving):**

Calories: 180.                    Protein: 3g

Carbohydrates: 20g.               Fat: 10g

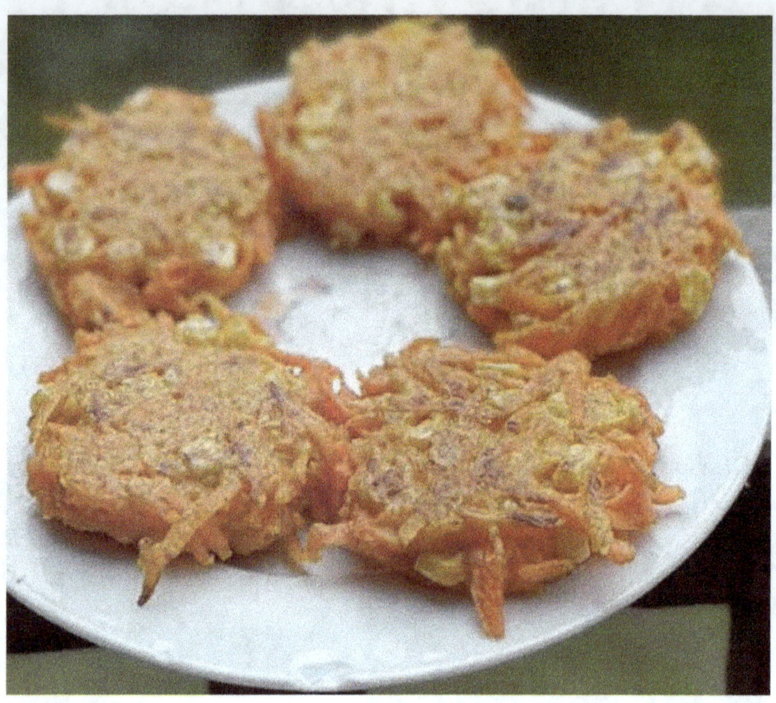

**Ingredients**:

- 1 cup sweetcorn kernels

- 1 cup carrots, grated

- 1/4 cup whole wheat flour

- 1 egg

- 1 teaspoon cumin

- Salt and pepper to taste

- 2 tablespoons olive oil (for cooking)

## Instructions:

1. In a bowl, combine sweetcorn, grated carrots, whole wheat flour, egg, cumin, salt, and pepper.

2. Heat olive oil in a pan and drop spoonfuls of the mixture.

3. Cook until fritters are golden on both sides.

## Alternative Ingredients:

Use whole wheat flour for added fiber.

Opt for egg whites to reduce cholesterol.

## Reasoning:

Whole wheat flour increases fiber content.

Egg whites reduce cholesterol and saturated fat.

## Nutritional Information (per serving):

Calories: 150.          Protein: 5g

Carbohydrates: 25g.     Fiber: 4g

Fat: 3g

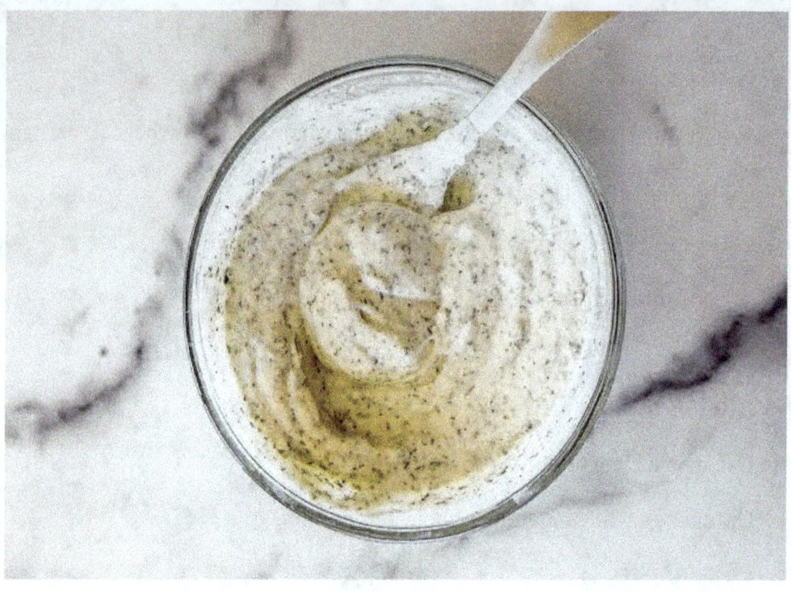

**Ingredients**:

- 1 cup fat-free Greek yogurt

- 1 teaspoon onion powder

- 1 teaspoon garlic powder

- 1 teaspoon dried dill

- 1 teaspoon dried parsley

- Salt and pepper to taste

**Instructions**:

1. Mix Greek yogurt, onion powder, garlic powder, dill, parsley, salt, and

pepper in a bowl.

2. Refrigerate before serving.


**Alternative Ingredients:**

Choose fat-free Greek yogurt for reduced fat.

Use fresh herbs like chives and parsley for added flavor.

Tips: Eat with any of your favourite snacks


**Reasoning:**

Fat-free Greek yogurt reduces overall fat content.

Fresh herbs enhance flavor without extra calories.


**Nutritional Information (per serving):**

Calories: 30

Protein: 2g

Carbohydrates: 4g

Fat: 0g

# 25. Strawberry FroYo

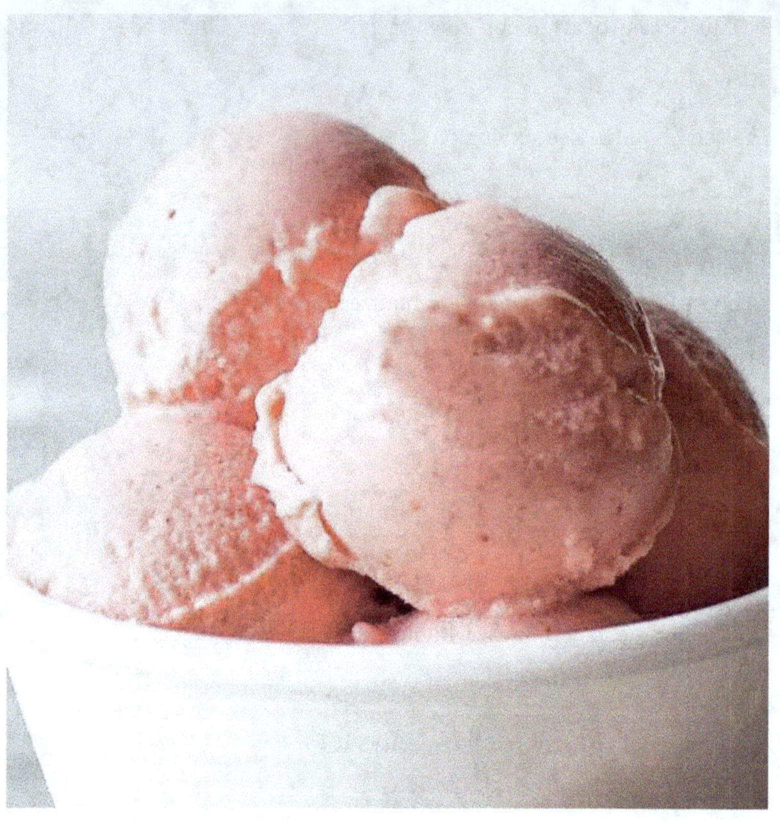

**Ingredients**:

- 2 cups frozen strawberries

- 1 cup fat-free Greek yogurt

- 1 tablespoon honey

- 1 teaspoon vanilla extract

**Instructions**:

1. Blend frozen strawberries, Greek yogurt, honey, and vanilla extract until smooth.

2. Serve immediately as a refreshing frozen yogurt.

**Alternative Ingredients:**

Opt for fat-free Greek yogurt for reduced fat.

Use a sugar substitute for sweetness.

**Reasoning:**

Fat-free Greek yogurt reduces overall fat content.

Sugar substitute cuts down on added sugars.

**Nutritional Information (per serving):**

Calories: 80

Protein: 6g

Carbohydrates: 15g

Fat: 0g

## 26. Weight Watchers Zero-Point Banana Souffle

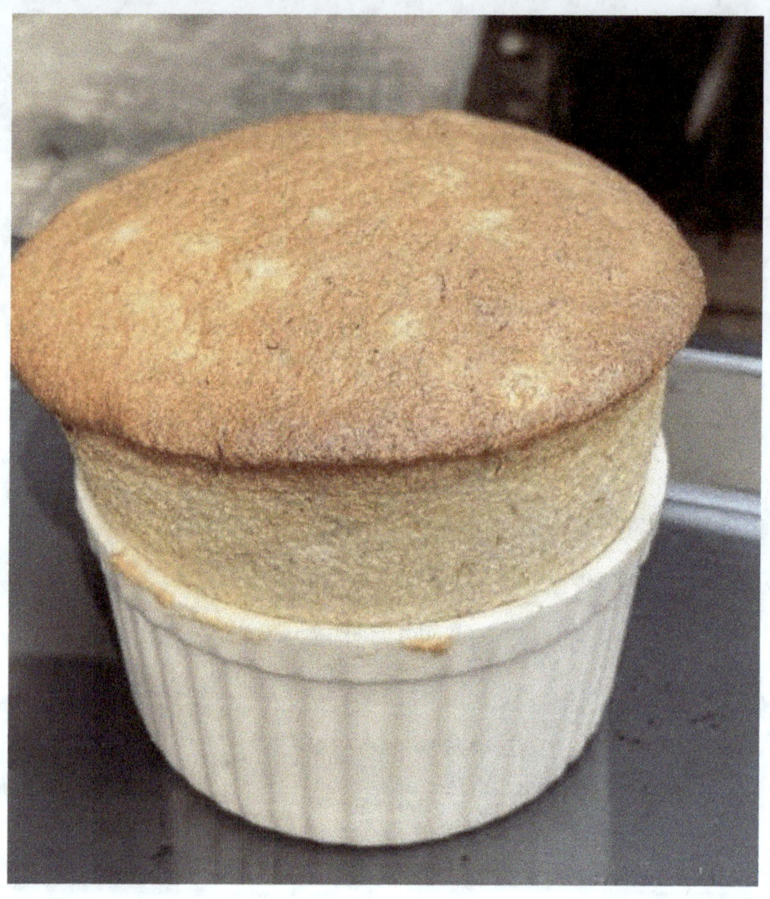

**Ingredients**:

- 3 ripe bananas, mashed

- 4 egg whites

- 1 teaspoon vanilla extract

- Pinch of salt

**Instructions**:

1. Preheat the oven to 375°F (190°C).

2. In a bowl, mix mashed bananas, egg whites, vanilla extract, and a pinch of salt.

3. Pour into individual ramekins.

4. Bake until soufflé is set and golden.

**Alternative Ingredients:**

Use egg whites instead of whole eggs for lower cholesterol.

Opt for almond milk for a dairy-free alternative.

**Reasoning:**

Egg whites reduce cholesterol and fat.

Almond milk provides a dairy-free option.

**Nutritional Information (per serving):**

Calories: 120

Protein: 5g

Carbohydrates: 25g

Fat: 1g

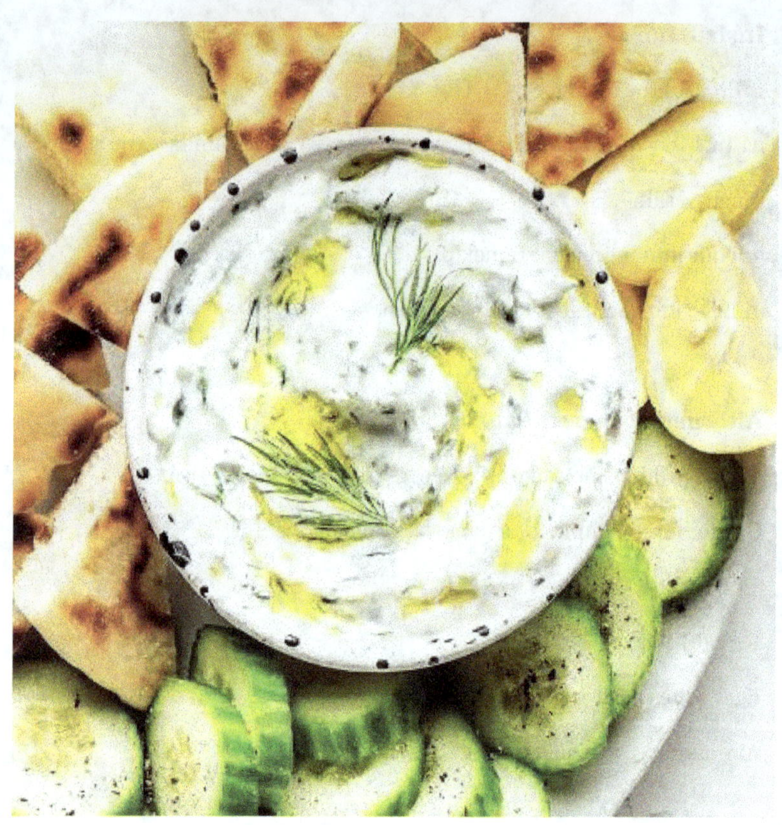

**Ingredients**:

- 1 cup fat-free Greek yogurt

- 1 cucumber, finely diced

- 2 cloves garlic, minced

- 1 tablespoon fresh dill, chopped

- 1 tablespoon lemon juice

- Salt and pepper to taste

**Instructions**:

1. In a bowl, combine Greek yogurt, cucumber, garlic, dill, lemon juice,

salt, and pepper.

2. Refrigerate before serving.

**Alternative Ingredients:**

Choose fat-free Greek yogurt for reduced fat.

Use fresh mint instead of dill for a different flavor.

**Reasoning:**

Fat-free Greek yogurt reduces overall fat content.

Fresh mint adds a unique flavor without extra calories.

**Nutritional Information (per serving):**

Calories: 25

Protein: 2g

Carbohydrates: 4g

Fat: 0g

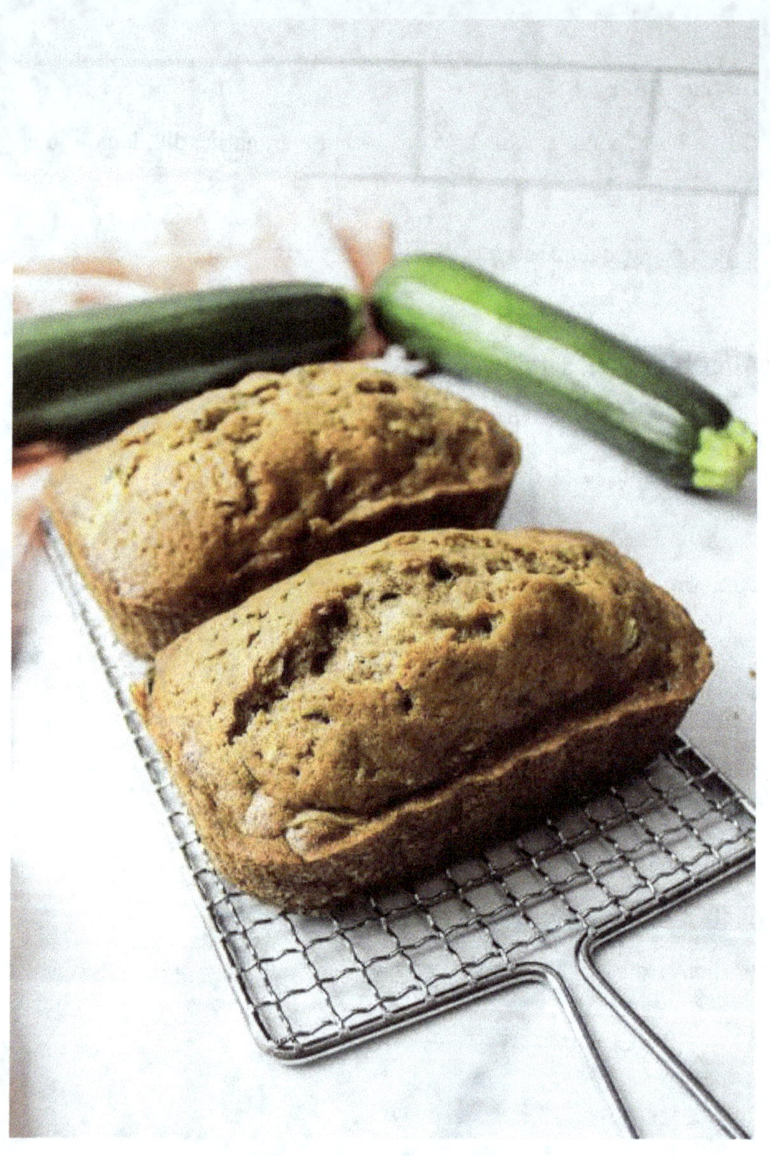

**Ingredients**:

- 2 cups grated zucchini

- 1/2 cup unsweetened applesauce

- 1/4 cup fat-free Greek yogurt

- 2 eggs

- 1 teaspoon vanilla extract

- 2 cups whole wheat flour

- 1 teaspoon baking powder

- 1/2 teaspoon baking soda

- 1 teaspoon cinnamon

- Pinch of salt

**Instructions**:

1. Preheat the oven to 350°F (175°C).

2. In a bowl, mix zucchini, applesauce, Greek yogurt, eggs, and vanilla extract.

3. In a separate bowl, whisk together whole wheat flour, baking powder, baking soda, cinnamon, and salt.

4. Combine wet and dry ingredients, then divide into mini loaf pans.

5. Bake until a toothpick comes out clean.

**Alternative Ingredients:**

Opt for whole wheat flour for added fiber.

Use unsweetened applesauce instead of oil for a lower-fat option.


**Reasoning:**

Whole wheat flour increases fiber content.

Unsweetened applesauce reduces fat content.


**Nutritional Information (per serving):**

Calories: 120

Protein: 3g

Carbohydrates: 20g

Fat: 3g

## 29. Roasted Pumpkin, Kale, and Couscous Salad

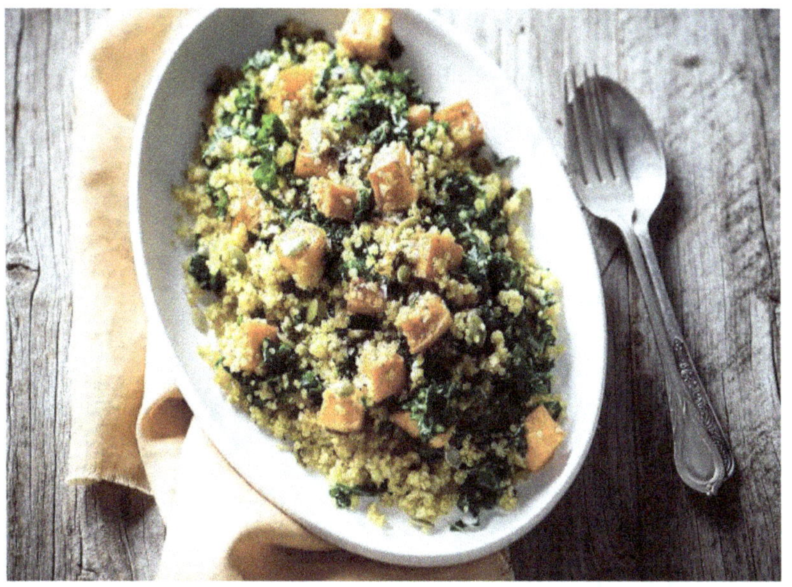

**Ingredients**:

- 2 cups pumpkin, diced

- 2 cups kale, chopped

- 1 cup whole wheat couscous, cooked

- 2 tablespoons balsamic vinegar

- 1 tablespoon olive oil

- Salt and pepper to taste

**Instructions**:

1. Preheat the oven to 400°F (200°C).

2. Toss pumpkin with olive oil, salt, and pepper; roast until tender.

3. Mix roasted pumpkin, kale, cooked couscous, and balsamic vinegar in a bowl.

**Alternative Ingredients:**

Choose quinoa instead of couscous for added protein.

Use balsamic vinaigrette made with olive oil for a heart-healthy dressing.

**Reasoning:**

Quinoa provides more protein and fiber than couscous.

Olive oil-based dressing adds healthy fats.

**Nutritional Information (per serving):**

Calories: 220

Protein: 6g

Carbohydrates: 40g

Fat: 5g

# 30. Curried Sausage Stew

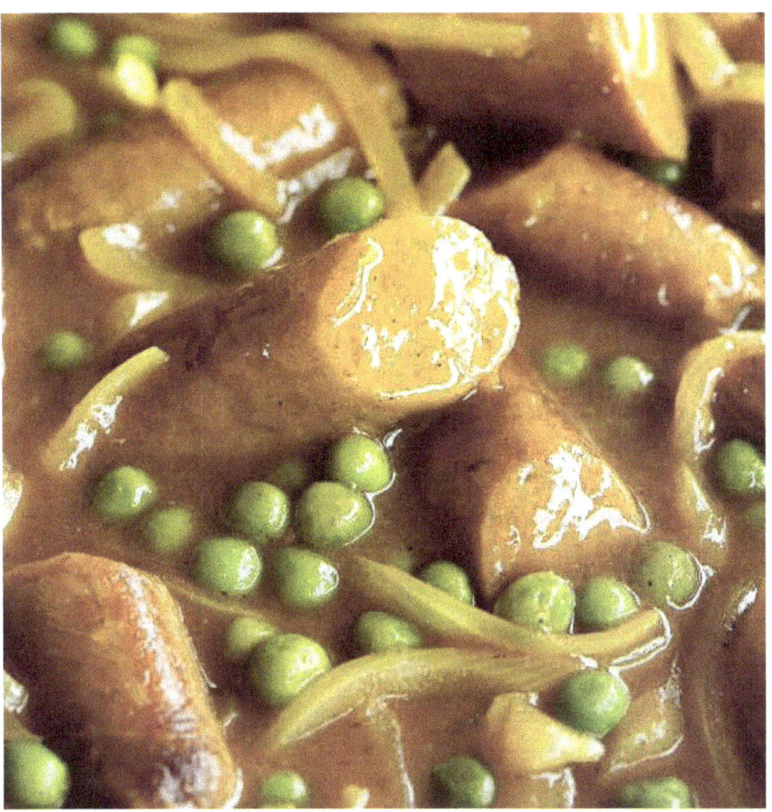

## Ingredients:

- 1 lb turkey or chicken sausage, sliced

- 1 onion, diced - 2 cloves garlic, minced

- 1 can (15 oz) diced tomatoes

- 1 can (15 oz) chickpeas, drained and rinsed

- 1 cup low-sodium chicken broth

- 1 tablespoon curry powder

- Salt and pepper to taste


**Instructions:**

1. In a pot, cook sausage until browned.

2. Add onion and garlic; cook until softened.

3. Stir in diced tomatoes, chickpeas, chicken broth, curry powder, salt, and pepper.

4. Simmer until flavors meld.


**Alternative Ingredients:**

Choose lean turkey or chicken sausage for lower fat content.

Opt for low-sodium vegetable broth to control sodium intake.


**Reasoning:**

Lean poultry sausage reduces saturated fat.

Low-sodium vegetable broth helps manage sodium levels.


**Nutritional Information (per serving):**

Calories: 250.                    Protein: 15g

Carbohydrates: 25g.               Fat: 10g

# 31. Lime Fluff

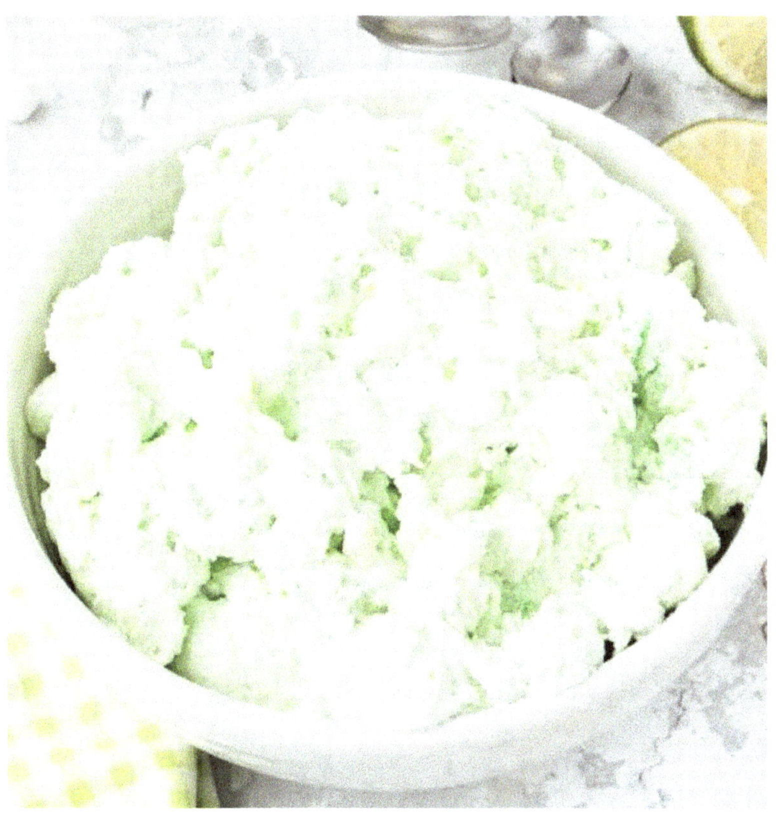

## Ingredients:

- 1 package sugar-free lime gelatin

- 1 cup fat-free cottage cheese

- 1 cup fat-free whipped topping

**Instructions**:

1. Prepare lime gelatin according to package instructions.

2. In a bowl, mix prepared gelatin, cottage cheese, and whipped topping.

3. Refrigerate until set.

**Alternative Ingredients:**

Use fat-free cottage cheese instead of regular for reduced fat.

Choose a sugar substitute for sweetness.

**Reasoning:**

Fat-free cottage cheese reduces overall fat content.

Sugar substitute decreases added sugars.

**Nutritional Information (per serving):**

Calories: 50

Protein: 5g

Carbohydrates: 10g

Fat: 0g

# 32. Cauliflower Crust Pizza with Veggie Toppings

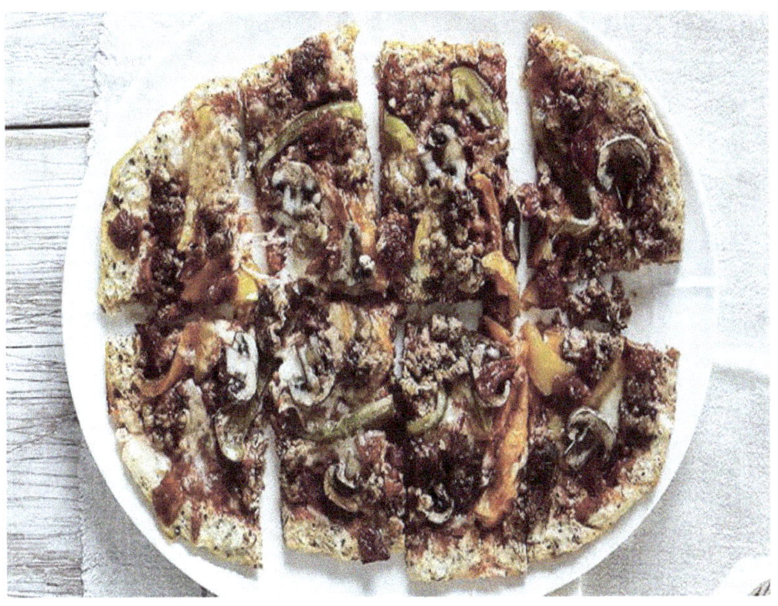

## Ingredients:

- 1 cauliflower head, grated

- 2 eggs

- 1/2 cup fat-free mozzarella cheese

- 1 teaspoon Italian seasoning

- Pizza sauce, veggies, and lean protein for toppings

## Instructions:

1. Preheat the oven to 400°F (200°C).

2. Mix grated cauliflower, eggs, mozzarella cheese, and Italian seasoning.

3. Spread mixture into a pizza shape and bake until edges are golden.

4. Add sauce, veggies, and protein as desired; bake until toppings are cooked.

**Alternative Ingredients:**

Opt for cauliflower rice in the crust for a lower-carb option.

Use a variety of colorful veggies for added nutrients.

**Reasoning:**

Cauliflower rice reduces carbohydrate content.

Colorful veggies boost nutritional value.

**Nutritional Information (per serving):**

Calories: 200

Protein: 10g

Carbohydrates: 15g

Fat: 10g

### 33. Weight Watchers Zero-Point Chocolate Mug Cake

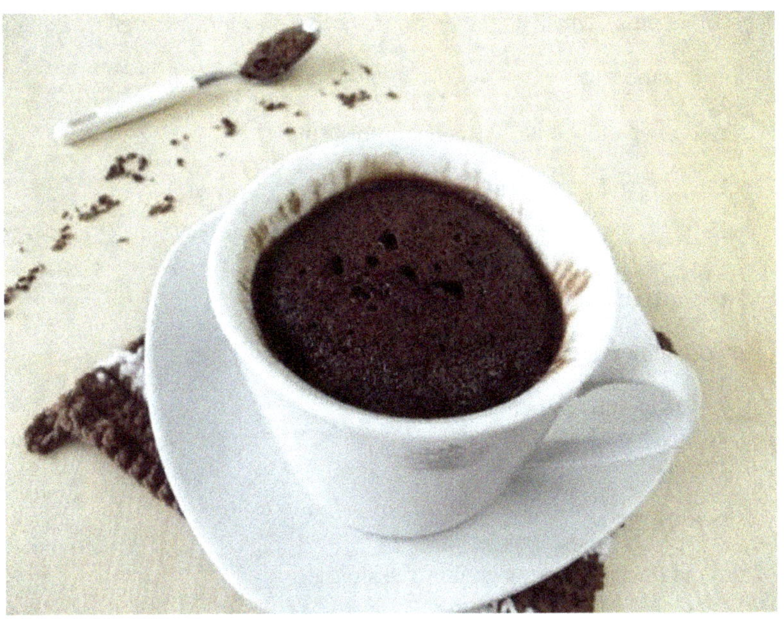

**Ingredients**:

- 3 tablespoons flour

- 2 tablespoons unsweetened cocoa powder

- 1 tablespoon sweetener (stevia or your preference)

- 1/4 teaspoon baking powder

- Pinch of salt

- 3 tablespoons fat-free milk

- 1/2 teaspoon vanilla extract

**Instructions**:

1. In a mug, whisk together flour, cocoa powder, sweetener, baking powder, and salt.

2. Add milk and vanilla extract; stir until smooth.

3. Microwave for 1-2 minutes until set.

**Alternative Ingredients:**

Choose almond flour for a gluten-free option.

Use a sugar substitute for sweetness.

**Reasoning:**

Almond flour provides a gluten-free alternative.

Sugar substitute reduces added sugars.

**Nutritional Information (per serving):**

Calories: 150

Protein: 7g

Carbohydrates: 15g

Fat: 8g

## 34. Easy Pasta Bake

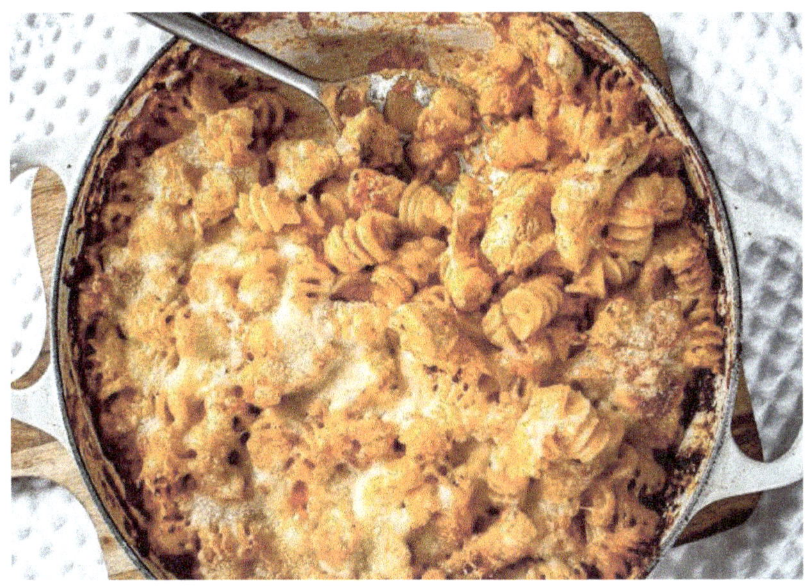

**Ingredients**:

- 8 oz whole wheat pasta, cooked

- 1 lb ground turkey or chicken

- 1 onion, diced

- 2 cloves garlic, minced

- 1 can (15 oz) tomato sauce

- 1 teaspoon Italian seasoning

- 1 cup fat-free mozzarella cheese, shredded

**Instructions**:

1. Preheat the oven to 375°F (190°C).

2. In a skillet, cook ground meat until browned.

3. Add onion and garlic; cook until softened.

4. Mix in cooked pasta, tomato sauce, and Italian seasoning.

5. Transfer to a baking dish, top with mozzarella, and bake until cheese is

melted.


**Alternative Ingredients:**

Opt for whole wheat pasta for added fiber.

Use lean ground turkey or chicken for a lower-fat option.


**Reasoning:**

Whole wheat pasta increases fiber content.

Lean ground turkey or chicken reduces saturated fat.


**Nutritional Information (per serving):**

Calories: 300

Protein: 20g

Carbohydrates: 35g

Fat: 10g